BREAKFAST SMOOTHIES

50 AMAZING RECIPES FOR WEIGHT LOSS AND START YOUR DAY HEALTHY

Amanda Smith

DISCLAIMER

A smoothie is a thick blend of fruits, vegetables, and dairy products that are rich in protein, minerals and vital supplements. You need a smoothie when you don't have time to make meals as it is a Mighty meal replacement that will fill your body with everything it needs on the go.

Who doesn't love smoothies? A whipped mixture of delicious and creamy ingredients will make you feel like you are top of the world.

So Be smart, learn to make a mind boggling smoothie from this ultimate smoothie cookbook and replace boring beverages with colorful and fast to make perfect smoothies.

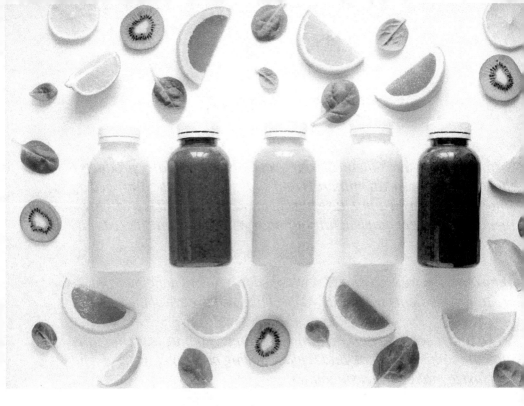

Table of contents

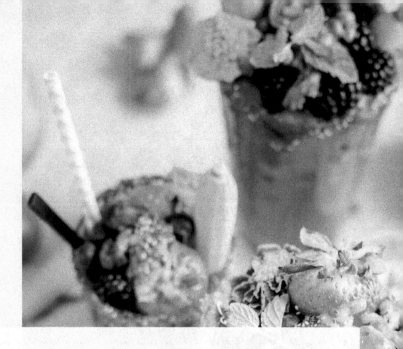

ALL YOU NEED TO KNOW ABOUT SMOOTHIES

"Add a sip of organic, healthy and happy delights to your dreams"

Smoothies are a thickened and blended version of a dairy beverage that has a similar consistency to a shake. They are the pureed form of various combinations of fruit juices, vegetable juices, milk, or even yoghurt. Some smoothies also have various protein powders, multivitamins and other supplements.

People have started consuming smoothies as a part of their meal or even as their meal replacement. Smoothies have now become a demand in the market and are used as an alternative for the replacement of lattes, cappuccinos and other coffee-based drinks.

BASIC COMPONENTS OF A SMOOTHIE

Preparing a smoothie is a diverse task as you may add the ingredients of your choice. But traditionally, most of the smoothies consist of four parts. These 4 parts are:

1. The very first component of a smoothie is a liquid that is considered the base of the smoothie. This base can be either, milk, coconut water or any fruit or vegetable juice.
2. The second component is an assortment of fruits and/or vegetables. These fruits or vegetables are preferably demanded to be frozen. On the other hand, fresh fruits and vegetables can also be used.
3. The third component is the ice that is a considerable component because it helps to retain the thick texture and consistency of the smoothie. Moreover, it enhances the taste of the smoothie as it chills it.
4. The fourth component is the garnishing item or sprinkles that can be either fruit or vegetable chunks being used in the smoothie, or some flavoured powder or sweet sauce.

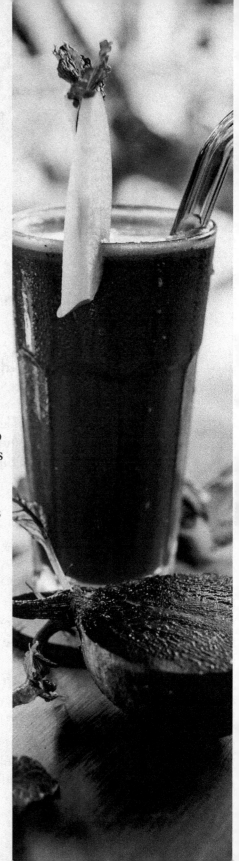

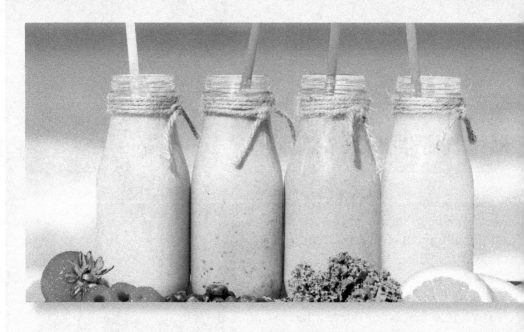

VARIOUS CATEGORIES OF SMOOTHIES

For almost 100 years, people have been making smoothies of their choice. This has led to the development of a variety of smoothies with various ingredients and the way of their preparation. The various recipes can be categorized as:

1. Fruit Smoothies:

These are the smoothies that are made from frozen or fresh fruits. The most popular fruit smoothies are berry smoothies, mango smoothies and banana smoothies. Fruits smoothies have their specificity of being sweet even without using any additional sweetener.

2. Green Smoothies:

Green smoothies are considered to be obtained from green vegetables that's why it is named so. The most popular green smoothies include Kale and spinach smoothie.

3. Nutritious and healthy Smoothies:

The smoothies that are prepared to target nutritional consent, is considered as a healthy smoothie. These smoothies provide the daily RDA of specific vitamins or minerals and aim to replace the supplements and medicines for a particular medical issue. Specific healthy smoothies can be heart-healthy, diabetic-friendly, protein-rich smoothies etc.

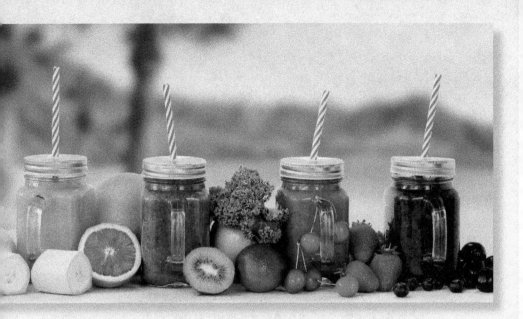

4. Weight Loss Smoothies:

The smoothie with a low glycemic index and no added sugars or sweeteners is the weight loss smoothie. They minimize the carb content and include healthy fats by adding flax seeds or almond butter that help the person to give the feeling of fullness. In weight loss smoothies, green tea, coffee or other caffeine-based stimulants can also be added that not only help to reduce the appetite but also improves the metabolism.

5. Confection Smoothies:

These smoothies are in the form of dessert and contain added sugar, artificial sweeteners and fats that are in the form of ice cream. The confection smoothies are dessert-like beverages having a taste similar to shakes.

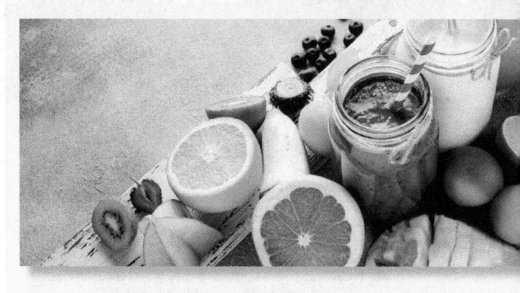

ARE SMOOTHIES PRIOR TO THE JUICES AND SHAKES?

Definitely yes!!
Smoothies contain non-processed, fresh, organic, fruits/vegetables and other items without any artificial sweeteners or syrups. Whereas, shakes contain a large number of processed sugars and ice-creams have been used while preparing the shakes.

On the other hand, juices are the concentrated form of fruits or vegetables and contain the left out juice only. While smoothies are blended mixtures of whole fruits and vegetables with all the original fibre content.

WHY DO YOU NEED SMOOTHIES?

Abundant reasons have convinced the essentiality of smoothies for our health as well as cravings. Smoothies being nutrient-dense, provide you with the maximum dietary intake of your nutritional needs. Despite being delicious and healthy, smoothies can also be a quick meal option with the right fuel for your energy.

Considerably, you need to add smoothies in your life because they can be your immunity and brain booster along with a sense of calm. Smoothies can be your life-changer if made with the right ingredients and using the recommended quantities.

Discussing the benefits of consuming smoothies in your diet will further elaborate its importance.

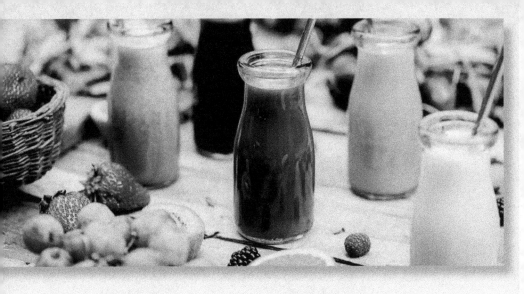

BENEFITS OF CONSUMING SMOOTHIES

1. GUT-FRIENDLY
Increased consumption of green leafy vegetables through the intake of smoothies aids in the digestion process. The high fibre content and the essential vitamins and minerals in these vegetables are the major contributors.

2. IMMUNITY BOOSTER
Smoothies have a good amount of beta-carotene that are helpful for the body to fight against pathogens and health conditions.

3. DETOXIFICATION
Several items like dandelion greens, kale, garlic, papaya and beets can cleanse the body thoroughly. The smoothies are helpful in the removal of toxins that are accumulated within the body tissues.

4. PREVENTS VARIOUS DISEASES
Specific smoothies are introduced to prevent or reduce the chance of a particular disease i.e. heart disease, diabetes, cancer, hypertension etc.

5. STRESS BUSTER
The fresh ingredients used for the preparation of smoothies contain the nutrients that not only boost your energy but also produce happy hormones. Smoothies can even control your mood swings and helps in fighting depression.

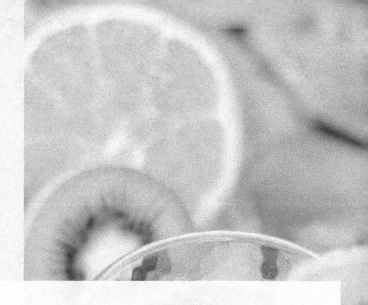

ARE SMOOTHIES HELPFUL IN THE WEIGHTLOSS?

Smoothies are the best option that can be helpful in your weight loss. Consuming an accurate smoothie with a proper lifestyle immensely reduces the weight. All you need is to create your perfect recipe that should be nutrient-dense with low caloric content.
Various kinds of weight loss smoothies have been introduced that provide adequate carbohydrates, proteins and fats while keeping the calories minimum.

The specific ingredients that are considered in the weight loss smoothie plan include chia seeds, flax seeds, avocados, nut butter and spinach. These ingredients create a feeling of fullness and help to lose weight. As per recent studies, it has also been proved that replacing a regular meal with any liquid form especially fruit/vegetable smoothie is beneficial to meltdown a few pounds.

BEAUTY BENEFITS OF SMOOTHIES

Clear skin and beauty glam is just a blender away!

All you need is a blender, some fruits or vegetables and a smoothie base. Blend them well and get clear glowy skin with mind-blowing results.
Smoothies contribute to the proper skin hydration with their anti-oxidant effect that makes you even younger and keeping the wrinkles away.
For this reason, researchers have developed a collagen-rich smoothie that helps you re-plenish the natural collagen supply of your body. It not only enhances the quality of the skin but also hair, nails, bones and joints. Raspberry smoothies and banana smooth-ies are considered helpful in the beauty benefits of skin. Moreover, papaya smooth-ie is a power fruit that helps clearing the skin pores as it.
contains essential vitamins. In addition to this, kale smoothie and coconut smoothie are for glowing and repairing skin.

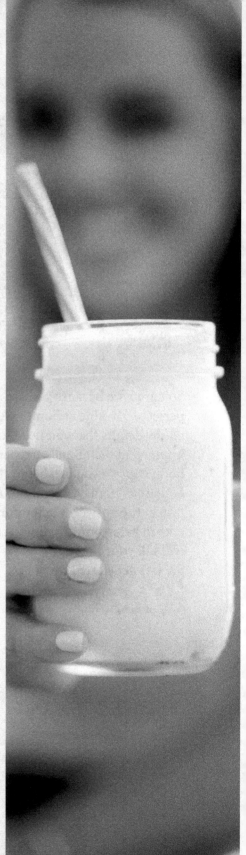

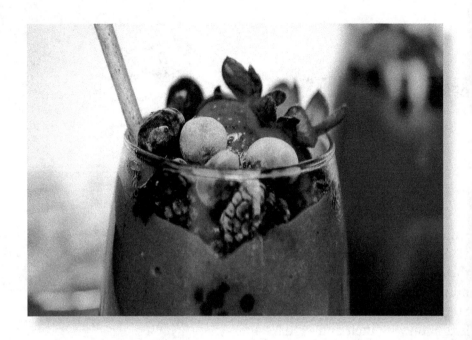

You are here because you are a smoothie lover and want to make a perfect smoothie at home. Well, ladies and gentlemen, you will get all the details that you need to know, from selecting the right tools to implement techniques, preparation guidelines, storage ideas, and some bonus tips so you can blend the perfect smoothie.

You are at home and want to make something delicious and nutritious, faster. The answer is smoothie; not only it will give you enough nutrients to help your immune system, brig flavour to your life and also it will kill your boredom.

So, let's get started.

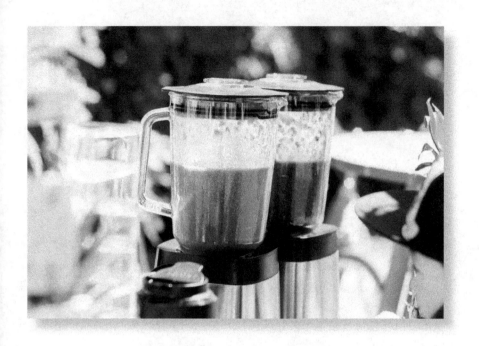

THE RIGHT KITCHEN TOOLS

To make a good smoothie, the first and foremost thing to do is to get the right kitchen tools. As you may already know that there is no better tool or equipment than a "Blender" to make a great smoothie. This smart piece of appliance machinery was invented in 1922 by Stephen J. Poplawski. Poplawski wanted to create something that can mix his fruits and vegetables into a go-to drink form and so he designed a blender by simply placing a spinning blade at the base of the glass container.

By the time of 1935, Frederick Osius and Fred Waring made major improvements on the fundamental design and then marketed it with the famous name of "Waring Blender." What happened next in the future was just history.

Talking about the structure and dimensions of a blender, it is made of metal, plastic, or more common glass material on top that is fitted with a stainless-steel blade at the base. Below the blades is the motor and chip integrated with the control panel that lets you control the speed of the rotary blades. It blends, chops, whips, and liquefies any crushable material you put in it. You can put something that is easily crushable, which means soft fruits, vegetables, and dry fruits. It is advised not to

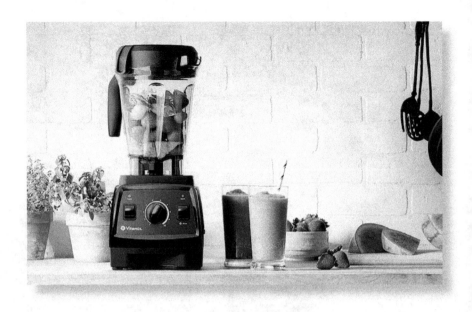

put something that is too hard so it doesn't harm the glass or mess up the blades.

Blender containers usually come in two distinct sizes: thirty-two ounces and forty ounces. If you are going to make smoothies for more than two or three people, choose a big-sized one.

Blender motors come in a variety of sizes. Those with 290-watt motors are good for most mixing operations, but not as good with smoothies. Some with 330 to 400 watts are considered to be professional and very good at crushing ice, a very important factor in creating excellent smoothies.

Blenders can be found in a variety of blade speed options, ranging from two-speed (high and low) to five and ten speeds. Variable-speed models offer many options, such as the ability to blend and whip.

CHOOSING A BLENDER

There are a variety of blender models on the market, and simply choosing a model randomly, or going with someone else's recommendations doesn't make much sense, because everyone has diverse needs and budgets.

This is where most people get really confused, so we have decided to take the challenge and make it as simple and easy as possible for you to choose a good blender that will last you for a long.

Just ask yourself what you would like to do with your blender.

That's why the first thing you need to do is to find a blender that you can be happy with for the long term. So, there are 4 main types of blenders that you should know about.

Each type has different goals and needs;

The main four types are: Hand Blenders, Traditional Countertop Blenders, Personal Bullet Blenders, and Top High-Performance Blenders.

1. Hand / Immersion Blenders

These are hand-held combinations, which often come with a variety of additives. This makes them more versatile and they can do every-thing from making soups and smoothies to marinades and even thick mayonnaise.

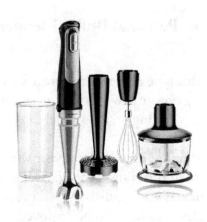

One of the great advantages of a hand blender is its compact size. If you have a small kitchen, this type of blender is the only one that does not take a huge space.

2. Countertop Blenders

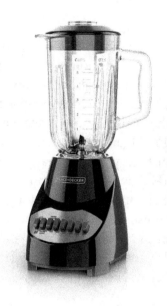

As you might have got the idea from the name, this type of blender is more likely to stay on your kitchen counter.

They are much stronger than hand blends but most of such models will not be able to cope with the wide range of smoothie ingredients as of bullet blenders or high-performance master chef style of smoothie blends.

3. Personal Bullet Blenders

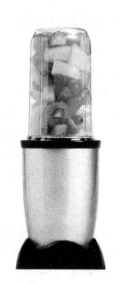

This type of blender is great for making one or two servings of smoothies (depending on the model).

They are usually slightly smaller than traditional jug-shaped blenders and have a 9mm bullet-shaped mixing glass cup that can be removed.

4. High-Performance Blenders

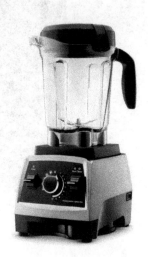

Simply put, this type of blender is the most powerful you can buy and is a Guru in dealing with the most challenging smoothie ingredients easily. The result - your smoothies will have a smooth and creamy texture that is a hallmark of that MasterChef type of blend.

Blendtec and Vitamix are some well-known blender names in this category, but there are also a few other blenders that have done a really good job, and it is up to you to buy the right one wisely.

Some factors that you must put into consideration before selecting any blender after choosing your category are to check the brand name and its history, price, durability, warranty, and by reading some reviews on the product, the decision making will become easy for you.

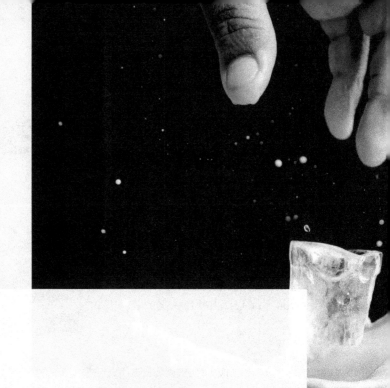

PREPARATION TIPS

Here are three methods or tips to prepare for your tasty smoothie before it is time to put the goodies in the blender's jug and rev up the blades.

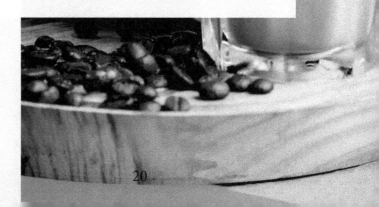

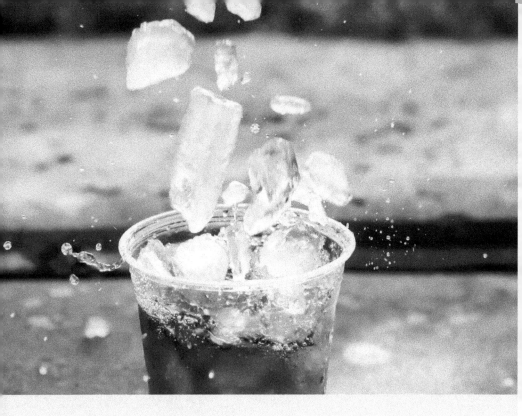

Tip 1: Ice cube tray method

The best way to make deliciously thick and cold smoothies ahead of time; because you can cherish the smoothie right away by simply crushing the ice cubes in your new blender.
What to do:
Once you have made your smoothies, pour them into an ice cube tray so that every "cube" space is evenly filled. For this, silicone trays are a good option as they are easily removable.

Place your ice tray in the deep freezer overnight, or you can make the material for up to a whole month.

When you are ready to get your favorite smoothie, put smoothie frozen cubes in a large glass-covered glass and transfer them to the refrigerator for about an hour. After that, give the glass a nice shake and that thick smoothie treat will be ready to consume!

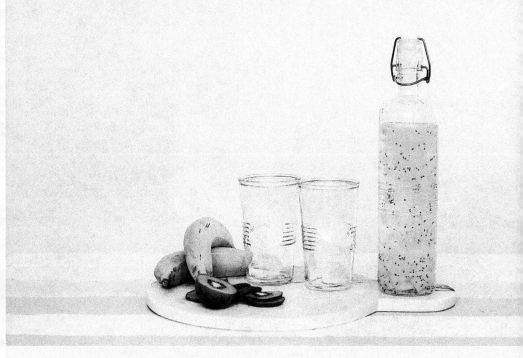

Tip 2: The glass jar technique

After you have made your smoothies to use for later on, simply buy a couple of mason jars and store the stuff in them.

You can store smoothies in that jar for as long as one month in the freezer and can simply consume them later on. Just take out the mason jar from the freezer a couple of hours before consuming or just take the frozen smoothie out at night and in the morning your smoothie breakfast will be ready

Tip 3: Wash your blender technique

Washing a dirty blender (and safely making sure the blades are clean) is both time-consuming and difficult. Just fill your dirty blender about halfway with water, add some dish soap, and turn the blender back on.

Then all you have to do is rinse away those bubbles and you're ready to make your next smoothie.

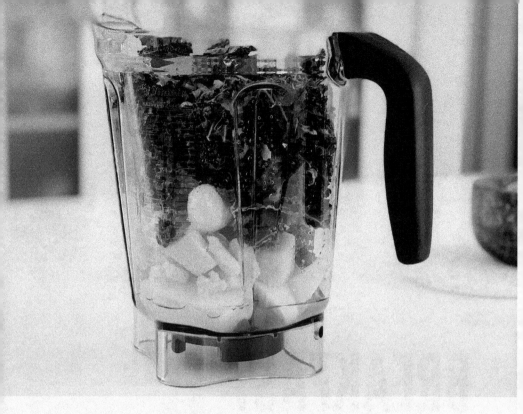

Some bonus tips to create better smoothies

- Try to read and research about different blends and trying out new taste combinations, trust me, it will never get boring this way.
- Buy a good quality blender, just don't fall for a cheap one. You may have to pay a little higher for a quality one but it will last you a lifetime and will make better blends.
- Try and make smoothies for at least a whole week and store them to consume quickly.
- Buy one with a removable glass top so you can clean it easily.

BREAKFAST
SMOOTHIES

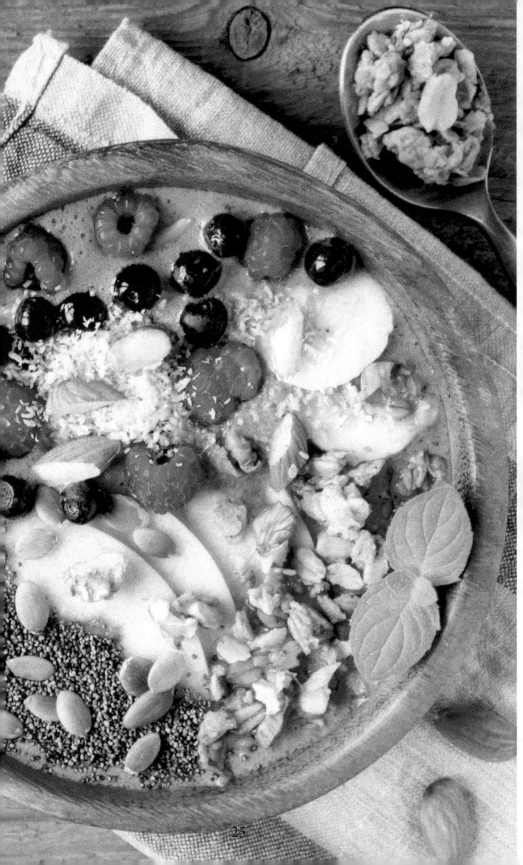

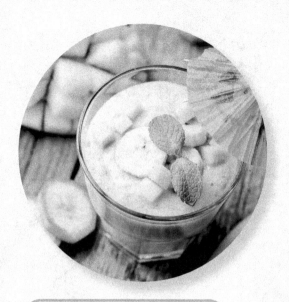

SUNRISE BREAKFAST SMOOTHIE

BREAKFAST SMOOTHIES

INGREDIENTS

- ½ cup frozen mango chunks
- ½ cup fresh pineapple chunks
- 1 frozen banana
- ¼ cup light coconut milk
- ¼ cup low-sugar orange drink, plus extra if desired
  1 cups plain non-fat yogurt
- Sliced bananas, fresh mango chunks, strawberries and fresh pineapple chunks

PREP TIME & SERVING

Prep time: 8 minutes
Total time: 8 minutes
Ready in about: 8 mins
No. of serve: 2

INSTRUCTIONS

01 Put the fruit, coconut milk and orange juice in a blender and blend until combined.

02 Add the yogurt to the blender and blend until smooth.

03 Add more orange juice to make the smoothie as thick as desired

04 Divide the smoothie into two glasses and top with sliced bananas, mango, strawberries and/or pineapple chunks.

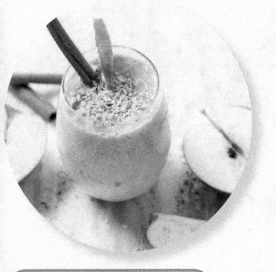

APPLE PIE SMOOTHIE

BREAKFAST SMOOTHIES

INGREDIENTS

- ½ cup old-fashioned un-cooked oats
- 1 cup plain Greek yogurt
- 1 medium-sized apple and pear
- ¼ cup milk or more if re-quired
- 1 teaspoon of cinnamon powder
- A pinch of ground nutmeg
- ¼ teaspoon vanilla extract
- 1 cup ice cubes

PREP TIME & SERVING

Prep time: 5 minutes
Total time: 10 minutes
Ready in about: 10 mins
No. of serve: 2

INSTRUCTIONS

01 Finely chop the uncooked oats in a blender. Add milk, apple, and pear to it.

02 In the end, add yogurt, cinnamon powder, nutmeg, and vanilla extract.

03 Make a smooth puree out of it by adding another tablespoon of milk if needed.Pulse the ice cubes in the blender.

04 Transfer the smoothie to a jar and sprinkle cinnamon powder to it.

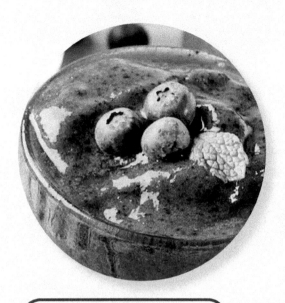

BLUEBERRY SMOOTHIE

BREAKFAST SMOOTHIES

INGREDIENTS

- 3 teaspoons old-fashioned oats
- 1 cup fresh spinach
- 1 cup frozen blueberries
- ¾ cup plain Greek yogurt
- ¾ cup milk (dairy or almond)
- 1/8 teaspoon cinnamon (Optional)

PREP TIME & SERVING

Prep time: 3 minutes
Total time: 5 minutes
Ready in about: 5 mins
No. of serve: 2

INSTRUCTIONS

01 Take a blender, add old-fashioned oats, and chopped.

02 Add milk (dairy or almond) of your choice, with blueberries and 1 cup fresh spinach.

03 In the end, add plain Greek yogurt and blend it all until it gives a smooth mixture.

04 Transfer the mixture into a smoothie jar and serve.

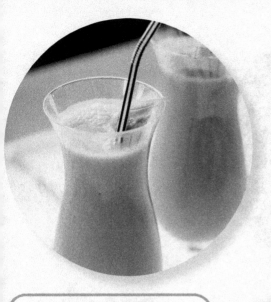

PUMPKIN SMOOTHIE

BREAKFAST SMOOTHIES

INGREDIENTS

- ¼ cup + 2 teaspoons old-fashioned oats
- ¼ cup canned pumpkin puree
- ¾ cup plain Greek yogurt
- 1 medium apple (peeled and pieces)
- ½ small frozen banana (sliced)
- ½ cup milk (dairy or almond
- 1/8 teaspoon pumpkin pie spice
- ½ cup ice cubes

PREP TIME & SERVING

Prep time: 5 minutes
Total time: 5 minutes
Ready in about: 5 mins
No. of serve: 2

INSTRUCTIONS

01 Firstly chopped oats in the blender.

02 Then add apple pieces, sliced banana, milk (dairy or almond), and yogurt.

03 In the end, add one teaspoon pumpkin pie spice together with pumpkin puree.

04 Blend all items with ice cubes and blend until it gives a smooth texture. Take a tall smoothie glass and pour the mixture and serve.

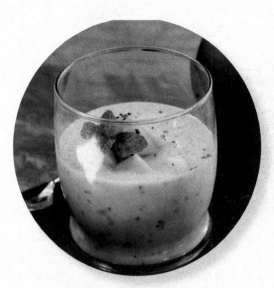

GREEN CHIA SEED SMOOTHIE

BREAKFAST SMOOTHIES

INGREDIENTS

- ½ cup frozen mango
- 1/3 cup Unsweetened almond milk
- 1 small orange, peeled
- 2 teaspoons chia seeds
- ¾ cup frozen pineapple chunks
- 1/3 small banana
- 1 cup loosely packed chopped kale

INSTRUCTIONS

01 In a blender adds frozen mango, chia seeds, and almond milk and pineapple chunks.

02 In the end adds rest items banana, peeled orange and chopped kale.

03 Blend the items until it gives a smooth texture.

04 Take a glass and pour the texture and serve.

PREP TIME & SERVING

Prep time: 5 minutes
Total time: 10 minutes
Ready in about: 10 mins
No. of serve: 2

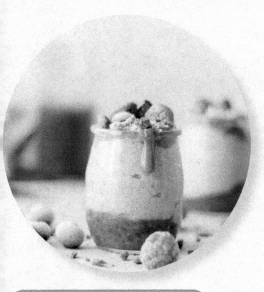

RASPBERRY PEANUT BUTTER SMOOTHIE

BREAKFAST SMOOTHIES

INGREDIENTS

- 1 ½ cups frozen raspberries
- 1 small banana
- 2 tablespoons peanut butter
- ¼ cup plain Greek yogurt
- Raspberries (fresh) to garnish
- 7 tablespoons ice water

INSTRUCTIONS

01 Grab a blender and adds small banana, peanut butter and Greek yogurt.

02 Now adds frozen raspberries in the end with ice water.

03 Blend all the ingredients well until it turns in a smooth mixture.

04 Top the mixture with more raspberries and serve with smoothie glass.

PREP TIME & SERVING

Prep time: 3 minutes
Total time: 5 minutes
Ready in about: 5 mins
No. of serve: 2

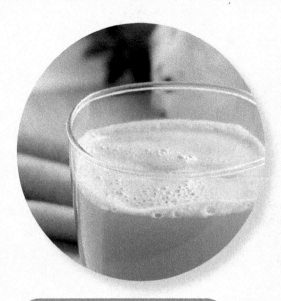

PINEAPPLE CARROT SMOOTHIE

BREAKFAST SMOOTHIES

INGREDIENTS

- 1 cup almond-coconut milk
- 4 tablespoons orange juice
- 1 cup frozen pineapple
- ½ banana
- 2 carrots (chopped and peeled)

PREP TIME & SERVING

Prep time: 5 minutes
Total time: 10 minutes
Ready in about: 10 mins
No. of serve: 2

INSTRUCTIONS

01 Take a high-speed blender and adds almond-coconut milk with frozen pineapple.

02 Adds banana and chopped carrots in the end and blend well.

03 Add orange juice one by one tablespoons during blending.

04 Give couples of minutes on blending to take a good consistency texture. Pour the texture in glass and serve.

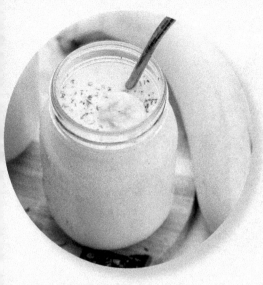

BANANA GREEK SMOOTHIE

BREAKFAST SMOOTHIES

INGREDIENTS

- 1 cup frozen sliced banana
- ¼ cup Greek yogurt
- ¼ cup milk (dairy or almond) your choice
- ¼ teaspoon vanilla extract

INSTRUCTIONS

01 Take a blender and adds frozen banana with Greek yogurt and vanilla extract.

02 Now adds milk and blend well if consistency is not according to your taste then add milk more.

03 When the mixture is smooth according to desire then pour in to glass and serve.

PREP TIME & SERVING

Prep time: 3 minutes
Total time: 5 minutes
Ready in about: 5 mins
No. of serve: 1

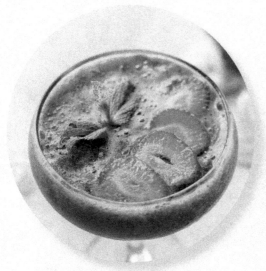

STRAWBERRY BANANA SMOOTHIE

BREAKFAST SMOOTHIES

INGREDIENTS

- 2 cups frozen strawberries
- 1 medium banana (fresh or frozen)
- ½ cup plain Greek yogurt, optional
- 1 cup milk (dairy or almond)

INSTRUCTIONS

01 Adds every ingredient in a blender and blend them well until it gives a best texture.

02 During the process use milk of your choice and adds yogurt as per your desire.

03 Pour the texture in glass and serve cooled.

PREP TIME & SERVING

Prep time: 5 minutes
Total time: 5 minutes
Ready in about: 5 mins
No. of serve: 1

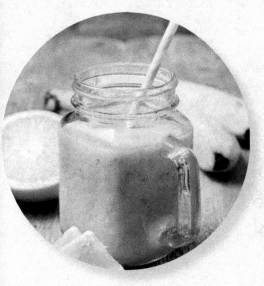

BOSSTING ORANGE SMOOTHIE

BREAKFAST SMOOTHIES

INGREDIENTS

- ½ medium banana
- 1 cup frozen mango slices
- ½ cup almond milk
- ¼ teaspoon vanilla extract
- 1 large orange(peeled)

INSTRUCTIONS

01 Grab a blender adds banana, peeled orange with mango slices.

02 Now adds almond milk and vanilla extract and blend them well.

03 When the mixture looks smooth then pour into glass and serve.

PREP TIME & SERVING

Prep time: 5 minutes
Total time: 5 minutes
Ready in about: 5 mins
No. of serve: 1

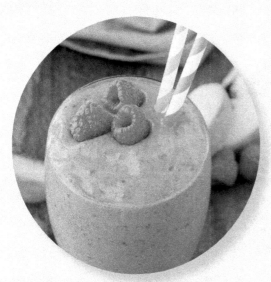

PEACH AND RASPBERRY SMOOTHIE

BREAKFAST SMOOTHIES

INGREDIENTS

- ¾ cup chopped fresh peach
- 1 cup frozen raspberries
- ¼ cup plain Greek yogurt
- 1/3 cup milk (of choice)
- 1 teaspoon honey

INSTRUCTIONS

01 Take strong blender adds fresh chopped peach with raspberries and blend.

02 Now adds milk (dairy or almond) with Greek yogurt in end.

03 If the mixture is too thick adds more milk. When the consistency according to taste.

04 Then pour the smooth mixture in jar and add honey to sweetness and serve.

PREP TIME & SERVING

Prep time: 7 minutes
Total time: 10 minutes
Ready in about: 10 mins
No. of serve: 1

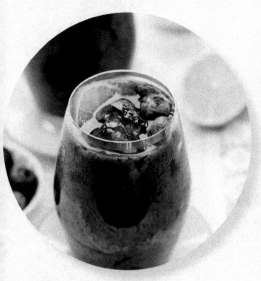

BLUEBERRY WITH COCONUT WATER

BREAKFAST SMOOTHIES

INGREDIENTS

- 1 cup coconut water
- 1 ½ cups frozen blueberries
- ½ cup yogurt full fat plain or Greek
- ¼ teaspoon coconut extract
- 1 tablespoon hemp hearts

INSTRUCTIONS

01 Add coconut water tighter with frozen blueberries in a speedy blender.

02 Now adds yogurt of your choice and hemp hearts and blend all of these.

03 Also add coconut extract in the end. When the texture looks smooth.

04 Pour the texture in smoothie jar and serve.

PREP TIME & SERVING

Prep time: 5 minutes
Total time: 10 minutes
Ready in about: 10 mins
No. of serve: 1

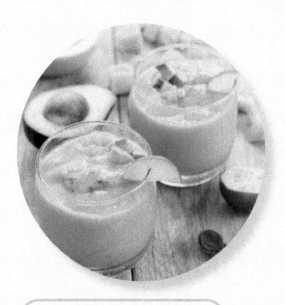

MANGO AVOCADO SMOOTHIE

BREAKFAST SMOOTHIES

INGREDIENTS

- 1 cup frozen mango chunks
- ½ banana frozen
- ½ cup ice cubes
- ½ -1 pineapple juice
- ½ cup Almond milk
- ¼ avocado
- Water place of milk (optional)

INSTRUCTIONS

01 Add all ingredients in a blender and blend well until it gives a smooth texture.

02 Use more juice of pineapple as your desire.

03 Pour the smooth mixture in a smoothie jar and serve.

PREP TIME & SERVING

Prep time: 3 minutes
Total time: 5 minutes
Ready in about: 5 mins
No. of serve: 1

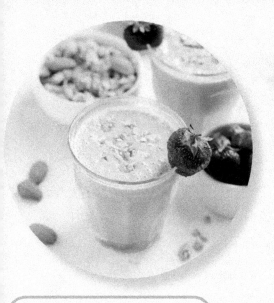

BEST BREAKFAST SMOOTHIE

BREAKFAST SMOOTHIES

INGREDIENTS

- 1 medium banana frozen
- 1 cup frozen strawberries
- 2 tablespoons rolled oatmeal
- ¼ cup vanilla protein powder
- 1 tablespoon peanut butter
- 1 cup almond milk

INSTRUCTIONS

01 Grab a blender adds rolled oatmeal, frozen banana, and frozen strawberries.

02 Add vanilla protein powder, peanut butter, and almond milk in the end.

03 Blend well all ingredients until it becomes smooth.

04 Take a smoothie jar pour in it and serve.

PREP TIME & SERVING

Prep time: 5 minutes
Total time: 10 minutes
Ready in about: 10 mins
No. of serve: 1

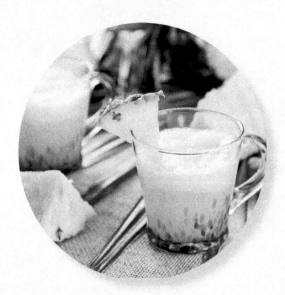

GINGER PINEAPPLE SMOOTHIE

BREAKFAST SMOOTHIES

INGREDIENTS

- 2 teaspoons fresh ginger or ground
- 1 cup frozen pineapple
- ½ medium banana
- ¼ cup Greek yogurt (low fat) or plain
- 1 teaspoon flax seed meal
- 1 cup fresh orange juice

INSTRUCTIONS

01 Grab a blender adds rolled oatmeal, frozen banana, and frozen strawberries.

02 Add vanilla protein powder, peanut butter, and almond milk in the end.

03 Blend well all ingredients until it becomes smooth.

04 Take a smoothie jar pour in it and serve.

PREP TIME & SERVING

Prep time: 3 minutes
Total time: 5 minutes
Ready in about: 5 mins
No. of serve: 1

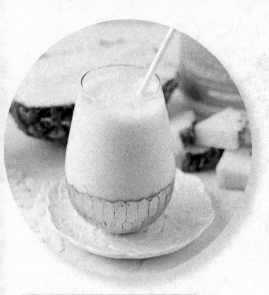

PINA COLADA SMOOTHIE

BREAKFAST SMOOTHIES

INGREDIENTS

- 2 cups frozen seasons fruits
- 1 cup coconut milk
- 1 teaspoon vanilla extract
- 1 tablespoon honey
- ½ cup fresh blueberries or pineapple chunks
- Coconut flakes and Millville oats (optional)

PREP TIME & SERVING

Prep time: 7 minutes
Total time: 10 minutes
Ready in about: 10 mins
No. of serve: 1

INSTRUCTIONS

01 Grab a high-speed blender and add frozen fruits with coconut milk and vanilla extract.

02 Now you can add fresh blueberries or pineapple chunks of your choice.

03 Add honey and coconut flakes in the end. Blend these entire well until it gives a smooth texture.

04 Take a smoothie glass and pour the mixture in it and toping with your optional ingredient and serve.

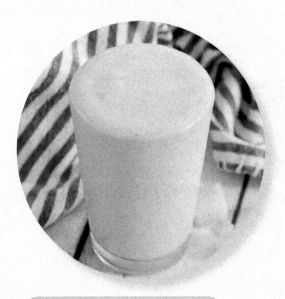

KEFIR SMOOTHIE

BREAKFAST SMOOTHIES

INGREDIENTS

- 1 large mango sliced
- 2 pieces of ginger
- ½ teaspoon ground turmeric
- ¾ cup fresh orange juice
- 1 cup kefir
- 1-2 tablespoon honey

INSTRUCTIONS

01 Take a high-speed blender to add mango, ground turmeric, and ginger.

02 Also, add the rest ingredients and blend them.

03 You can use more ginger, honey, and turmeric according to your taste.

04 When the mixture looks smooth; pour into the smoothie jar and serve.

PREP TIME & SERVING

Prep time: 5 minutes
Total time: 10 minutes
Ready in about: 10 mins
No. of serve: 1

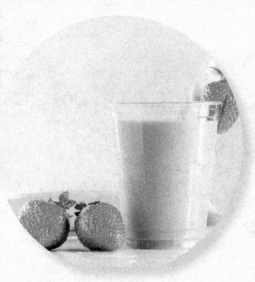

STRAWBERRY PROTINE SMOOTHIE

BREAKFAST SMOOTHIES

INGREDIENTS

- 1 ½ cups frozen strawberries
- ½ frozen banana
- ¼ cup vanilla protein powder of any kind
- 1 cup almond milk
- For topping crushed graham crackers

INSTRUCTIONS

01 Grab a blender add frozen strawberries, banana, and vanilla protein powder.

02 Also, add milk in the end and blend well until it gives a smooth mixture.

03 Pour the mixture into jar top crushed graham crackers and serve.

PREP TIME & SERVING

Prep time: 7 minutes
Total time: 10 minutes
Ready in about: 10 mins
No. of serve: 1

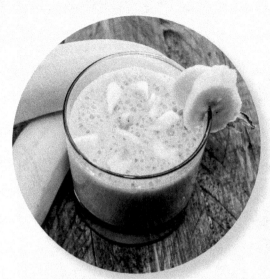

EASY QUICK SMOOTHIE

BREAKFAST SMOOTHIES

INGREDIENTS

- 1 banana
- 1 tablespoon porridge oats
- 80g soft fruits (of your choice)
- 150ml milk (dairy or almond)
- 1 teaspoon honey
- 1 teaspoon vanilla extract.

INSTRUCTIONS

01 Grab a blender, and add all entire ingredients and blend for a couple of minutes.

02 Blend well until it gives a smooth texture.

03 Pour the smoothie into a jar and serve.

PREP TIME & SERVING

Prep time: 3 minutes
Total time: 5 minutes
Ready in about: 5 mins
No. of serve: 1

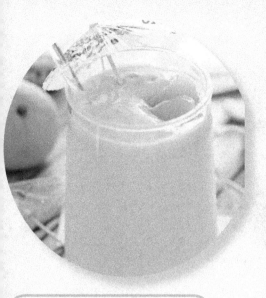

SUNSHINE SMOOTHIE

BREAKFAST SMOOTHIES

INGREDIENTS

- 1 ½ cups carrot juice chilled
- ¾ cup fresh pineapple chunks
- 2 frozen bananas
- 1 small piece of ginger
- 3 tablespoons cashew nuts
- 1 lime juice

INSTRUCTIONS

01 Take a blender, and add the entire ingredients and blend until it gives a smooth mixture.

02 Pour the texture into a smoothie jar and served.

PREP TIME & SERVING

Prep time: 5 minutes
Total time: 10 minutes
Ready in about: 10 mins
No. of serve: 1

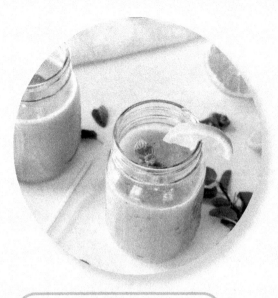

LEMON TURMERIC SMOOTHIE

BREAKFAST SMOOTHIES

INGREDIENTS

- 1 cup water
- 1 cup milk (dairy or almond)
- 1 lemon juice
- ½ teaspoon turmeric ground
- ¼ teaspoon ginger ground
- Pinch of cinnamon
- 1 teaspoon honey

INSTRUCTIONS

01 Grab a high-speed blender adds entire ingredients and blend well until it looks smooth mixture.

02 Add honey to the mixture as your required taste and pour in a glass and serve.

PREP TIME & SERVING

Prep time: 7 minutes
Total time: 10 minutes
Ready in about: 10 mins
No. of serve: 1

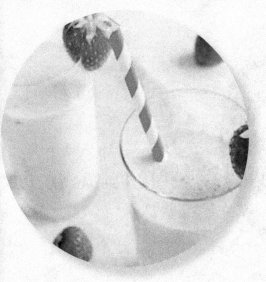

RUTH BERRY SMOOTHIE

BREAKFAST SMOOTHIES

INGREDIENTS

- 1 cup strawberries
- ½ cup pineapple
- 1 banana
- 2 cup orange juice
- ½ cup Greek yogurt
- 1 teaspoon chia seeds
- ½ cup ice cubes

INSTRUCTIONS

01 Take a high-speed blender adds orange juice, pineapple, and Greek yogurt.

02 Now add the rest ingredients and blend until it looks smooth.

03 Pour the mixture into a jar and serve.

PREP TIME & SERVING

Prep time: 5 minutes
Total time: 10 minutes
Ready in about: 10 mins
No. of serve: 1

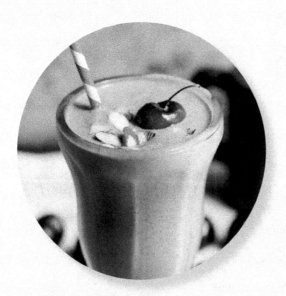

CHERRY ALMOND SMOOTHIE

BREAKFAST SMOOTHIES

INGREDIENTS

- 1 ½ cups cherries frozen
- 1 cup almond milk
- 1 tablespoon protein powder
- 1 banana
- ½ cup ice cubes
- Almond butter (optional)

INSTRUCTIONS

01 Use a high-speed blender; add frozen cherries, almond milk, and banana in the blender.

02 Also, add the rest ingredients and blend for a couple of minutes or until it gives a smooth texture.

03 Then pour the texture into the jar and serve.

PREP TIME & SERVING

Prep time: 5 minutes
Total time: 10 minutes
Ready in about: 10 mins
No. of serve: 1

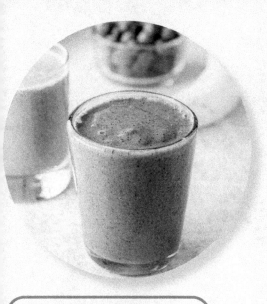

POWER HOUSE SMOOTHIE

BREAKFAST SMOOTHIES

INGREDIENTS

- 1 cup coconut milk
- 1 scoop chocolate protein powder
- ½ cup blueberries
- 1 cup spinach
- 1 banana
- 1 tablespoon almond butter
- 1 cup ice cubes

INSTRUCTIONS

01 Grab a blender adds the entire ingredients and blend until it looks smooth.

02 If it looks too thick then add more milk to attain the desired consistency.

03 Then pour the mixture into the jar and serve.

PREP TIME & SERVING

Prep time: 5 minutes
Total time: 10 minutes
Ready in about: 10 mins
No. of serve: 1

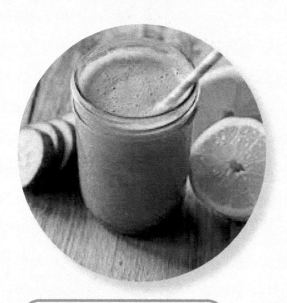

YOUTHFUL GLOW SMOOTHIE

BREAKFAST SMOOTHIES

INGREDIENTS

- 1 cup kale
- 1 cup baby spinach
- 1 cup pure apple juice
- ½ Cucumbers
- 2 tablespoon lemon juice
- I frozen banana
- ½ cup ice cubes
- 1 teaspoon fresh grated ginger

INSTRUCTIONS

01 Take a high-speed blender adds the rest ingredients and blend until it gives a mixture.

02 Use grated ginger as your desired (optional) and pour the mixture in a smoothie jar and serve.

PREP TIME & SERVING
Prep time: 5 minutes
Total time: 10 minutes
Ready in about: 10 mins
No. of serve: 1

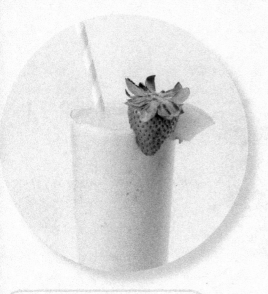

BREAKFAST SMOOTHIES

INGREDIENTS

- 1 cup frozen raspberries
- ½ cup frozen mango
- ½ cup frozen pineapple
- 1 cup coconut milk or dairy milk

INSTRUCTIONS

01 Add desire milk with raspberries, frozen mango, and frozen pineapple in a blender.

02 Blend until it gives a smooth texture, pour it into a smoothie jar and serve.

PREP TIME & SERVING

Prep time: 5 minutes
Total time: 10 minutes
Ready in about: 10 mins
No. of serve: 1

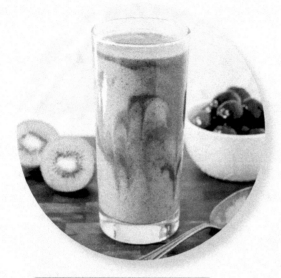

SUPERDARK SMOOTHIE

BREAKFAST SMOOTHIES

INGREDIENTS

- 1 cup frozen cherries
- 1 whole kiwi
- 1 cup almond milk
- 1 tablespoon chia seeds

INSTRUCTIONS

01 Blend entire ingredients frozen cherries, kiwi with milk, and chia seeds in a blender.

02 Blend until it looks creamy and smooth then pour it into a jar and serve.

PREP TIME & SERVING

Prep time: 5 minutes
Total time: 10 minutes
Ready in about: 10 mins
No. of serve: 1

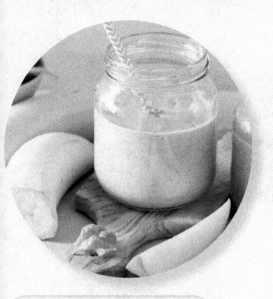

BREAKFAST SMOOTHIES

INGREDIENTS

- 2 tablespoon lemon juice
- 1 large frozen banana
- 1 cup frozen mango chunks
- 1 ½ cups baby Spinach

INSTRUCTIONS

01 Grab a high-speed blender and add lemon juice, banana, mango, and baby spinach to blend.

02 When the mixture looks smooth then pour it into the jar and serve.

PREP TIME & SERVING

Prep time: 5 minutes
Total time: 10 minutes
Ready in about: 10 mins
No. of serve: 1

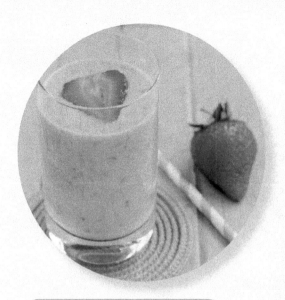

DAYDREAM SMOOTHIE

BREAKFAST SMOOTHIES

INGREDIENTS

- ½ cup frozen peaches
- 1 cup plain yogurt
- ½ cup coconut water
- 1 cup frozen strawberries

INSTRUCTIONS

01 Take a high-speed blender and add all the ingredients in it.

02 Blend until it gives a smooth mixture.

03 Pour the smooth mixture into jar and serve.

PREP TIME & SERVING

Prep time: 5 minutes
Total time: 10 minutes
Ready in about: 10 mins
No. of serve: 1

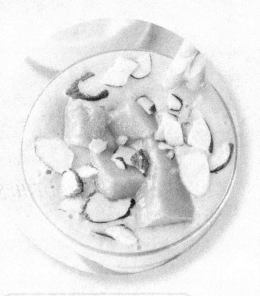

MANGO BREAKFAST SMOOTHIE

BREAKFAST SMOOTHIES

INGREDIENTS

- 1 cup almond milk
- 1 frozen banana
- ½ cup frozen mango
- 1-2 baby spinach
- ¼ cup pumpkin seeds
- 2 tablespoons hemp heart seeds
- 2 tablespoons vanilla protein powder
- ¼ cup of water

INSTRUCTIONS

01 Grab high-powered blender add almond milk together with banana, mango, and baby spinach,

02 Also, add the rest ingredients and blend well until it gives a smooth texture.

03 Pour the texture into the jar and serve.

PREP TIME & SERVING

Prep time: 5 minutes
Total time: 10 minutes
Ready in about: 10 mins
No. of serve: 1

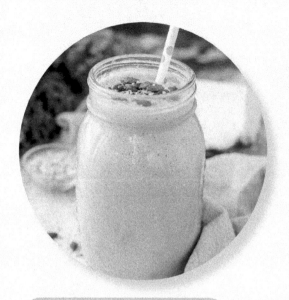

CREAMY SMOOTHIE

BREAKFAST SMOOTHIES

INGREDIENTS

- 1 cup kale chopped
- 1 ½ cup frozen pineapple chunks
- ½ cup Greek yogurt
- ½ cup almond milk
- 1 teaspoon honey

PREP TIME & SERVING

Prep time: 3 minutes
Total time: 5 minutes
Ready in about: 5 mins
No. of serve: 1

INSTRUCTIONS

01 Grab a strong blender and add chopped kale, pineapple chunks with almond milk.

02 Add the rest ingredients into the blender and blend until it looks smooth.

03 Add honey according to your taste.

04 Take a glass and pour the mixture in it and serve.

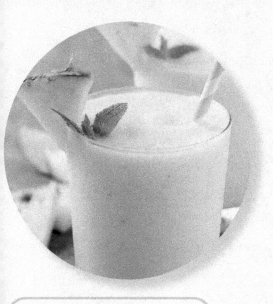

CITRUS-PINEAPPLE SMOOTHIE

BREAKFAST SMOOTHIES

INGREDIENTS

- ½ cup Greek yogurt (low fat)
- ½ cup frozen pineapple
- 1 teaspoon vanilla extract
- ½ cup orange juice
- ½ ruby grapefruit
- 1 tablespoon chia seeds, coconut flaks (optional)

INSTRUCTIONS

01 Use a high-speed blender and add low-fat Greek yogurt together with frozen pineapple.

02 Add vanilla extract, grapefruit, and orange juice.

03 Blend all of these ingredients for a couple of minutes.

04 When the texture looks smooth then pour it into the glass jar.

05 Top it with your optional ingredient and serve.

PREP TIME & SERVING

Prep time: 3 minutes
Total time: 5 minutes
Ready in about: 5 mins
No. of serve: 1

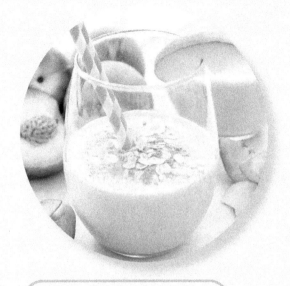

CREAMY PEACHES OATMEAL SMOOTHIE

BREAKFAST SMOOTHIES

INGREDIENTS

- ½ cup full fat milk
- ½ cup Greek yogurt
- ½ cup rolled oats
- 1 cup frozen peaches
- 1 medium frozen banana
- ½ cup ice cubes

INSTRUCTIONS

01 Add all the ingredients in a speedy blender.

02 Blend the ingredients until it gives a smooth texture.

03 If its consistency is too thick then add more milk or yogurt.

04 When your mixture looks then pour it into the smoothie glass and serve.

PREP TIME & SERVING

Prep time: 5 minutes
Total time: 10 minutes
Ready in about: 10 mins
No. of serve: 1

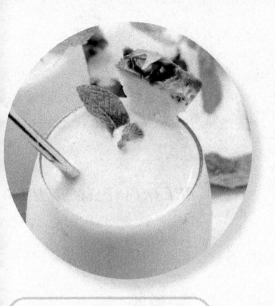

PASSION BREAKFAST SMOOTHIE

BREAKFAST SMOOTHIES

INGREDIENTS

- 1 cup vanilla yogurt
- 6 ice cubes
- 1 cup pineapple chunks

INSTRUCTIONS

01 Add every ingredient in a blender and pulse until it gives smooth texture.

02 Then pour it into the jar and serve.

PREP TIME & SERVING

Prep time: 3 minutes
Total time: 5 minutes
Ready in about: 5 mins
No. of serve: 1

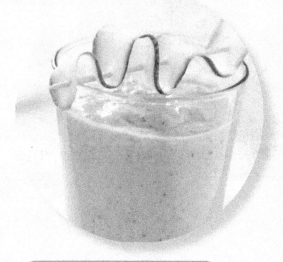

MILK AND HONEY SMOOTHIE

BREAKFAST SMOOTHIES

INGREDIENTS

- 1 ½ cups almond milk
- 1 medium Kirby cucumber
- 1 cup green grapes (seedless)
- 2 medium stalks celery
- 1 tablespoon

INSTRUCTIONS

01 Grab a blender and add almond milk together with green grapes and cucumber.

02 In the end add the rest ingredients and pulse well.

03 When mixture looks smooth then add honey according to your taste.

04 Then pour the smoothie into the jar and serve.

PREP TIME & SERVING

Prep time: 5 minutes
Total time: 10 minutes
Ready in about: 10 mins
No. of serve: 1

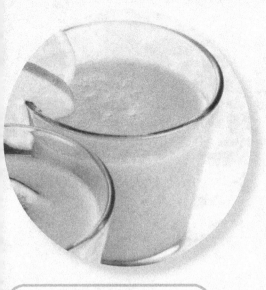

SILKY SKIN SMOOTHIE

BREAKFAST SMOOTHIES

INGREDIENTS

- ½ cup ice cubes
- ½ cup full fat Greek yogurt.
- ¼ cup grated carrot
- 1 tablespoon honey
- ½ teaspoon cinnamon
- 2 chopped dried apricots
- 1 fresh apricot (pitted and chopped)

INSTRUCTIONS

01 In a blender add the ice cubes with milk, carrot, and yogurt.

02 Finely add the remaining ingredients to the blender.

03 Blend them until it turns in a smooth texture.

04 Pour the texture into a smoothie bowl and serve.

PREP TIME & SERVING

Prep time: 7 minutes
Total time: 10 minutes
Ready in about: 10 mins
No. of serve: 1

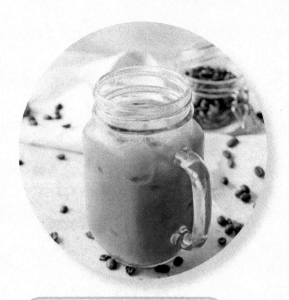

ICE COFFEE SMOOTHIE

BREAKFAST SMOOTHIES

INGREDIENTS

- 1 cup strong brewed coffee, cooled
- 1/2 cup reduced-fat (2%) milk
- 1 tablespoons sugar
- 1 tablespoon light chocolate syrup
- 1 cup ice cubes

INSTRUCTIONS

01 Combine the ingredients in a blender and blend until smooth.

02 Pour the mixture into the smoothie glass and serve.

PREP TIME & SERVING

Prep time: 4 minutes
Total time: 4 minutes
Ready in about: 4 mins
No. of serve: 2

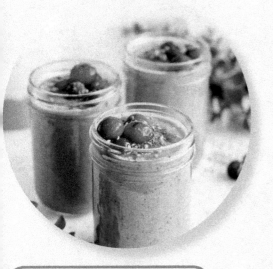

CRANBEREY SMOOTHIE

BREAKFAST SMOOTHIES

INGREDIENTS

- 1 cup frozen cranberries
- 1 cup almond milk
- 1 medium banana
- 1 tablespoon maple syrup
- ½ cup ice cubes

INSTRUCTIONS

01 Grab a blender and add frozen cranberries, almond milk, and banana.

02 Now add maple syrup, and ice cubes in the end.

03 Blend all these ingredients well until it gives a smooth texture.

04 Take a glass and pour the texture into the glass and serve.

PREP TIME & SERVING

Prep time: 5 minutes
Total time: 7 minutes
Ready in about: 7 mins
No. of serve: 1

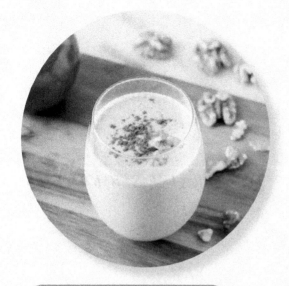

APPLE PIE SMOOTHIE

BREAKFAST SMOOTHIES

INGREDIENTS

- 1 cup apple cider
- ½ cup vanilla Greek yogurt
- ¼ old-fashioned rolled oats
- 2 tablespoon pecans
- ¼ teaspoon cinnamon
- ¼ teaspoon nutmeg
- 1 cup ice cubes

PREP TIME & SERVING

Prep time: 5 minutes
Total time: 10 minutes
Ready in about: 10 mins
No. of serve: 1

INSTRUCTIONS

01 Take a high-speed blender and add Greek yogurt, rolled oats, and ice cubes.

02 Now add the entire ingredients in it and blend for a couple of minutes.

03 If it doesn't look smooth then blend for more some time.

04 When it gives smooth mixture then pour it into the smoothie glass.

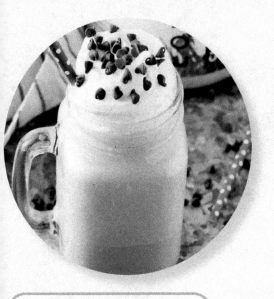

MOCHA PROTIEN SMOOTHIE

BREAKFAST SMOOTHIES

INGREDIENTS

- 1 ½ cup black coffee
- 1 large banana
- 1 cup ice cubes
- ¼ cup walnuts
- 1 tablespoon cocoa powder
- 6 tablespoon chocolate powder

INSTRUCTIONS

01 Grab a high-speed blender and add the entire ingredients.

02 Blend them until it looks smooth mixture.

03 Then pour the mixture in a smoothie jar and serve.

PREP TIME & SERVING

Prep time: 5 minutes
Total time: 10 minutes
Ready in about: 10 mins
No. of serve: 1

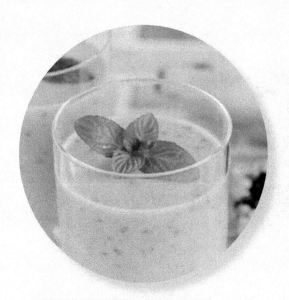

PAPAYA PERFECTION SMOOTHIE

BREAKFAST SMOOTHIES

INGREDIENTS

- 1 cup papaya chunks
- 1 cup plain yogurt (low fat)
- ½ fresh pineapple chunks
- ½ cup ice cubs
- 1 teaspoon coconut extract
- 1 teaspoon ground flax seeds

INSTRUCTIONS

01 Blend papaya chunks with fat-free plain yogurt.

02 Then add pineapple chunks and the entire ingredients into the blender.

03 Blend them until it gives smooth mixture then pour it into the glass and serve.

PREP TIME & SERVING

Prep time: 5 minutes
Total time: 10 minutes
Ready in about: 10 mins
No. of serve: 1

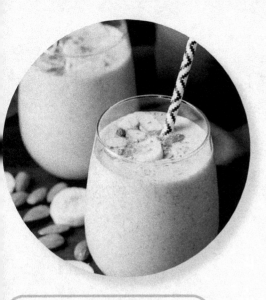

BANANA ALMOND SMOOTHIE

BREAKFAST SMOOTHIES

INGREDIENTS

- ½ cup coconut water
- ½ cup plain Greek yogurt
- 3 tablespoon almond butter
- 1 scoop whey protein powder
- 1 tablespoon hemp seeds
- 1 frozen banana
- 1 cup ice cubes

INSTRUCTIONS

01 Grab a blender and add coconut water, almond butter, and Greek yogurt.

02 Now add protein powder, hemp seed, and banana, with ice cubes.

03 Blend all these entire ingredients well until it looks smooth texture.

04 Then pour the texture in a glass and serve.

PREP TIME & SERVING

Prep time: 5 minutes
Total time: 10 minutes
Ready in about: 10 mins
No. of serve: 1

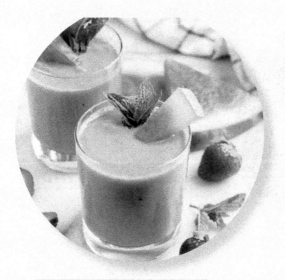

WATERMELON WONDER SMOOTHIE

BREAKFAST SMOOTHIES

INGREDIENTS

- 2 cups chopped watermelon
- ¼ cup milk (dairy or almond)
- 2 cups ice cubes

INSTRUCTIONS

01 Add watermelon, and milk of your choice with ice cubes in a blender.

02 Blend them until it turns in a smooth mixture.

03 Then pour the mixture in a smoothie jar and serve.

PREP TIME & SERVING

Prep time: 5 minutes
Total time: 10 minutes
Ready in about: 10 mins
No. of serve: 1

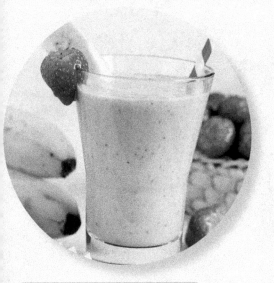

TUTTI-FRUTTI SMOOTHIE

BREAKFAST SMOOTHIES

INGREDIENTS

- ½ cup frozen berries of your choice
- ½ cup canned pineapple chunks
- ½ cup plain yogurt
- ½ cup sliced banana
- ½ cup orange juice

INSTRUCTIONS

01 Take a blender and add all entire ingredients in it.

02 Blend them for a couple of minutes or until the mixture turns in smooth.

03 Then pour it into the jar and serve.

PREP TIME & SERVING

Prep time: 5 minutes
Total time: 10 minutes
Ready in about: 10 mins
No. of serve: 1

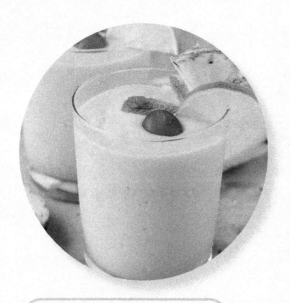

MANGO MADNESS SMOOTHIE

BREAKFAST SMOOTHIES

INGREDIENTS

- 1 cup frozen vanilla yogurt (fat-free)
- 1 mango
- 1 banana
- 1 canned pineapple chunks
- 1 cup of ice cubes

INSTRUCTIONS

01 Put all the ingredients into a blender and blend until it turns to a smooth and creamy mixture.

02 Pour this mixture into a jar.

03 Top it with more pineapple chunks and serve.

PREP TIME & SERVING

Prep time: 5 minutes
Total time: 7 minutes
Ready in about: 7 mins
No. of serve: 1

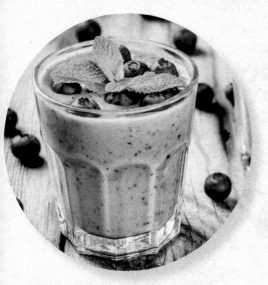

JUMP-START SMOOTHIE

BREAKFAST SMOOTHIES

INGREDIENTS

- 1 cup fresh orange juice
- 1 cup frozen strawberries
- ½ cup fresh blueberries
- 2 teaspoon fresh ginger
- ¼ cup low fat plain yogurt
- ½ cup ice cubes

INSTRUCTIONS

01 Take a strong blender and add the entire ingredients in it.

02 Blend them for a couple of minutes.

03 When it gives a smooth texture then pour it into glass and serve.

PREP TIME & SERVING
Prep time: 5 minutes
Total time: 5 minutes
Ready in about: 5 mins
No. of serve: 1

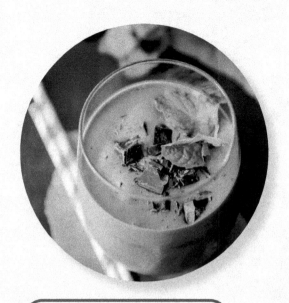

MINT CHOCOLATE SMOOTHIE

BREAKFAST SMOOTHIES

INGREDIENTS

- ½ of an avocado
- ¼ cup vanilla Greek yogurt
- ¼ cup chocolate protein powder
- 1 tablespoon honey
- ¼ teaspoon peppermint extract
- ¾ cup milk dairy or almond
- ½ cup baby spinach
- ½ cup ice
- 1 tablespoon chocolate chips (for topping)

INSTRUCTIONS

01 Grab a high-speed blender and add milk of your choice and avocado with baby spinach.

02 Now add peppermint extract, honey, and chocolate powder with ice cubes in the end.

03 Blend them well until it turns into a smooth mixture.

04 Then pour it into the glass and top it with chocolate chips and serve.

PREP TIME & SERVING

Prep time: 5 minutes
Total time: 5 minutes
Ready in about: 5 mins
No. of serve: 1

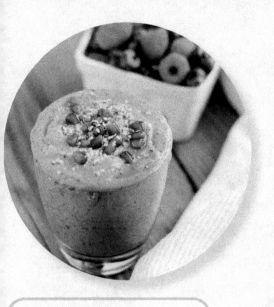

POMEGRANATE-BERRY SMOOTHIE

BREAKFAST SMOOTHIES

INGREDIENTS

- ½ cup chilled pomegranate juice
- ½ cup vanilla yogurt low-fat
- 1 cup frozen mixed berries

INSTRUCTIONS

01 Take a strong blender and add all entire ingredients in it.

02 Blend them until it gives a smooth form.

03 Then pour it into the smoothie jar and serve.

PREP TIME & SERVING

Prep time: 5 minutes
Total time: 5 minutes
Ready in about: 5 mins
No. of serve: 1

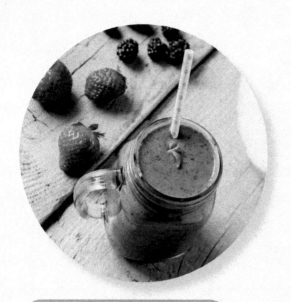

GRAPEFRUIT BREAKFAST SMOOTHIE BOWL

BREAKFAST SMOOTHIES

INGREDIENTS

- ¼ cup grapefruit juice
- 1 frozen banana
- ½ tablespoon honey
- ½ cup frozen strawberries
- 4 ice cubes

Toppings
- Sliced fresh strawberries
- Sliced grapefruit
- Sliced banana
- Sliced blackberries

INSTRUCTIONS

01 Add frozen banana, strawberries, honey, grapefruit juice, and ice cubes into a blender and blend until smooth.

02 If the mixture is thick, then add more ice until it reaches the desired consistency.

03 Pour smoothie into a bowl and garnish with the sliced fresh strawberries, grapefruit, banana, and blackberries.

PREP TIME & SERVING

Prep time: 5 minutes
Total time: 5 minutes
Ready in about: 5 mins
No. of serve: 1

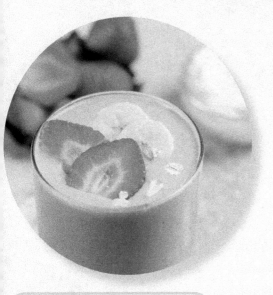

FRUIT AND YOGURT BREAKFAST SMOOTHIE

BREAKFAST SMOOTHIES

INGREDIENTS

- 1 banana, peeled
- ½ cup low-fat plain yogurt
- 1 cup orange juice
- ½ cup strawberries
- ½ cup ice cubes

INSTRUCTIONS

01 Take a blender, add banana, orange juice, strawberries, yogurt, and ice cubes blend until smooth.

02 When it looks smooth, then pour into two glasses. Serve fresh.

PREP TIME & SERVING

Prep time: 5 minutes
Total time: 5 minutes
Ready in about: 5 mins
No. of serve: 1

CPSIA information can be obtained
at www.ICGtesting.com
Printed in the USA
BVHW090816280521
608293BV00005B/1776